HAIR CARE @ HOME

DIY SOLUTIONS FOR COMMON PROBLEMS

DR MUKESH AGGARWAL

Contents

Preface

Welcome to the world of self-care and empowerment through hair care! This book is a passport to understanding, nurturing, and celebrating the incredible crown of strands we call our hair.

In today's fast-paced world, we often overlook the simple yet profound art of caring for our locks at home. Hair, beyond being a reflection of beauty, is a canvas of individuality, expressing our personalities and embracing our uniqueness.

This guide is not just a collection of remedies; it's a journey through the fascinating world of homegrown solutions for seven common hair dilemmas. From the persistent battle against hair loss to the quest for that elusive shine and the age-old challenge of premature greying, each chapter unravels the secrets and remedies to reclaiming your hair's vitality.

But this book is more than just solutions. It's an ode to the holistic approach of nurturing hair—where lifestyle changes, proper nutrition, natural remedies, and a touch of mindfulness converge to create a harmonious relationship between you and your tresses.

As we delve into this world of hair care, let's embark on a transformative journey—one that not only rejuvenates our hair but also revitalizes our self-confidence and connection with our own unique beauty.

So, let's dive in, explore, experiment, and, most importantly, discover the joy of caring for our hair at home.

With love,
Dr. Mukesh Aggarwal

Acknowledgements

Creating this comprehensive guide on DIY hair care wouldn't have been possible without the support, guidance, and contributions from numerous individuals and sources. I extend my heartfelt gratitude to:

My family, whose unwavering support and encouragement fueled my passion for holistic health and wellness.

The tireless efforts of my colleagues and peers who shared their invaluable insights and experiences in the realm of hair care.

The readers and supporters who inspire me to continue exploring and sharing knowledge in the pursuit of healthier lifestyles.

The countless ancient wisdom traditions and modern research that have shaped and enriched our understanding of holistic hair care practices.

The team behind the scenes—editors, designers, and everyone involved in bringing this book to life.

Last but not least, to every individual committed to embracing and nurturing their hair's natural beauty. Your curiosity and dedication to self-care inspire me endlessly.

Your collective contributions and unwavering support have made this endeavor a reality. Thank you for being an integral part of this journey toward healthier, happier hair.

With gratitude,
Dr. Mukesh Aggarwal

Introduction

The Importance of Home Hair Care

Hair, often referred to as one's crowning glory, holds immense significance in our lives. Beyond aesthetics, healthy hair contributes to our confidence and overall well-being. Therefore, understanding the importance of home hair care is crucial in maintaining its health and vitality.

Firstly, regular hair care routines at home are essential to upkeep hair health. Simple practices like regular washing with a suitable shampoo and conditioner help to remove dirt, oil, and environmental pollutants that accumulate in the hair. This routine aids in maintaining a clean scalp, preventing issues like dandruff or infections.

Moreover, proper hydration is key. Just as our body needs hydration, so does our hair. Adequate water intake, along with the use of moisturizing hair products, ensures that hair remains hydrated and less prone to dryness and breakage.

Additionally, the significance of using appropriate hair products cannot be overstated. Different hair types require different care. Understanding one's hair type helps in choosing the right products, whether it's for moisturizing curly hair, adding volume to fine hair, or controlling frizz in thick hair.

Furthermore, the use of heat styling tools necessitates caution. Excessive heat exposure can lead to damage and weaken the hair shaft. Therefore, using heat protectants and minimizing heat exposure helps in safeguarding the hair's integrity.

Notably, a balanced diet plays a crucial role in maintaining healthy hair. Nutrients like protein, vitamins, and minerals are fundamental for hair growth and strength. Incorporating a diet rich in these nutrients promotes healthier hair from within.

Lastly, establishing a consistent routine is paramount. Consistency in caring for one's hair yields better results over time. Developing a regular schedule for washing, conditioning, and treating the hair ensures its continual upkeep.

In conclusion, the importance of home hair care cannot be overlooked. Through regular maintenance, appropriate product selection, and a healthy lifestyle, one can ensure that their hair remains healthy, vibrant, and a source of confidence and pride.

BRIEF OVERVIEW OF COMMON HAIR PROBLEMS

Hair serves as a significant aspect of our identity and self-expression. However, numerous challenges often plague our quest for healthy and vibrant hair. Understanding these common hair problems is crucial in adopting suitable strategies to address and overcome them.

Hair Loss, a prevalent concern for many, manifests in various forms. Whether it's gradual thinning, receding hairlines, or bald patches, hair loss can stem from genetics, hormonal imbalances, stress, nutritional deficiencies, or underlying health conditions. Seeking professional guidance aids in determining the root cause and potential treatments for this distressing issue.

Dandruff, characterized by itching and flaking, affects countless individuals. This scalp condition results from factors such as dry skin, a yeast-like fungus called Malassezia, sensitivity to hair products, infrequent shampooing, or an imbalance in scalp oils. Incorporating medicated shampoos, maintaining good scalp hygiene, and addressing potential triggers can help manage and alleviate dandruff.

Dryness and Damage pose common challenges to hair health. Excessive heat styling, chemical treatments, over-washing, exposure to harsh weather elements, and inadequate moisture contribute to dry, brittle hair prone to breakage and split ends. Nourishing hair with deep conditioning treatments, reducing heat exposure, and adopting protective hairstyles can revitalize and strengthen damaged hair.

Oily or Greasy Hair stems from overactive sebaceous glands, resulting in excess oil production. Genetics, hormonal fluctuations, or washing hair too frequently can contribute to this issue. Balancing oil production through proper hair care routines, using clarifying shampoos, and avoiding excessive manipulation of the scalp can help manage greasy hair.

Frizzy Hair presents as unruly, unmanageable strands that stand out due to their rough texture. Factors such as humidity, lack of moisture, damage, or genetic predisposition contribute to this problem. Utilizing anti-frizz products, deep conditioning, and protective styling techniques aid in taming frizz and restoring a smoother texture.

Scalp Infections, caused by bacterial or fungal agents, result in redness, itching, tenderness, and sometimes hair loss. Poor hygiene, compromised immunity, or exposure to contaminated surfaces contribute to these infections. Seeking medical attention for proper diagnosis and treatment is crucial to alleviate scalp infections.

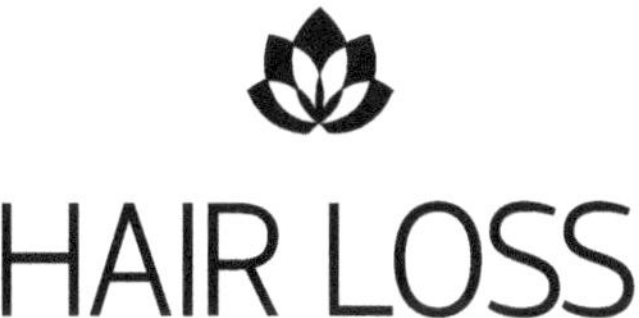

CHAPTER ONE

HAIR LOSS

TYPES OF HAIR LOSS

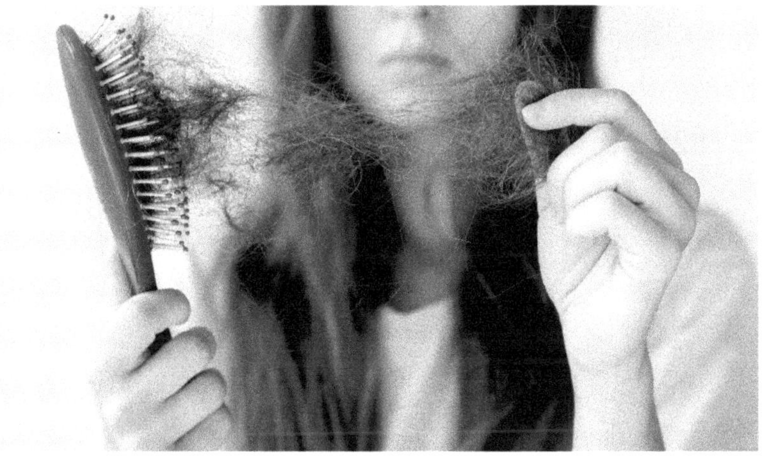

Fig. 1.1 Image showing excessive hair loss

Androgenetic Alopecia: Commonly known as male or female pattern baldness, it's the most prevalent type, influenced by genetics and hormonal changes. It results in a receding hairline or thinning on the crown.

Alopecia Areata: This is an autoimmune condition causing patchy hair loss on the scalp or body due to the immune system attacking hair follicles.

Telogen Effluvium: Triggered by stress, illness, surgery, or hormonal changes, it leads to a widespread thinning of hair across the scalp due to a disruption in the hair growth cycle.

Traction Alopecia: Caused by repeated pulling or tension on the hair follicles, common in hairstyles like tight braids, ponytails, or extensions.

Nutritional Deficiencies: Inadequate intake of essential nutrients like iron, zinc, or protein can lead to hair loss.

Causes of Hair Loss

Genetics: Androgenetic alopecia is often inherited from either parent and is associated with hormonal changes.

Hormonal Changes: Imbalances due to pregnancy, childbirth, menopause, or thyroid disorders can contribute to hair loss.

Medical Conditions: Scalp infections, autoimmune diseases like lupus, and other health issues can cause hair loss.

Stress: Physical or emotional stress can trigger telogen effluvium, leading to excessive shedding of hair.

Certain Medications: Some drugs used for cancer, arthritis, depression, heart problems, and high blood pressure can cause hair loss as a side effect.

Poor Hair Care Practices: Excessive use of heating tools, harsh chemical treatments, tight hairstyles, or improper hair care routines can damage hair and lead to loss.

Understanding the type of hair loss and its underlying cause is essential for proper management and treatment. Seeking advice from a healthcare professional or a dermatologist can provide personalized solutions to mitigate or address the issue effectively.

HOME REMEDIES FOR PREVENTING HAIR LOSS

Hair loss can be distressing, but several natural remedies can help in preventing it or slowing it down. These remedies focus on nourishing the scalp, strengthening hair follicles, and promoting a healthy environment for hair growth.

1. Scalp Massage: Regular scalp massages with essential oils like coconut, almond, or castor oil can improve blood circulation, stimulate hair follicles, and reduce hair fall. This encourages hair growth and strengthens the roots.

2. Aloe Vera: Known for its healing properties, aloe vera gel applied directly to the scalp can soothe and condition it. It helps balance the pH levels, reducing dandruff and promoting healthy hair growth.

3. Onion Juice: High in sulfur, onion juice aids in improving blood circulation to hair follicles, reducing inflammation, and promoting hair regrowth. It's applied to the scalp and left for about 30 minutes before rinsing.

4. Egg Mask: Rich in proteins and biotin, eggs help strengthen hair strands. A mixture of eggs and olive oil, applied as a mask and rinsed after 20 minutes, can nourish the hair and prevent breakage.

5. Balanced Diet: A diet rich in vitamins, minerals, and proteins is crucial for healthy hair. Including foods like nuts, seeds, leafy greens, eggs, fish, and fruits can provide essential nutrients for hair growth.

6. Green Tea: Applying cooled, brewed green tea to the scalp can help in preventing hair loss. It contains antioxidants that support hair health by reducing damage and promoting growth.

7. Fenugreek Seeds: Soaking fenugreek seeds overnight and grinding them into a paste can be applied to the scalp to reduce hair fall and encourage hair growth.

8. Hibiscus Flower: A paste made from hibiscus flowers and leaves can nourish the hair, prevent dryness, and encourage growth when applied to the scalp.

9. Avoiding Harsh Treatments: Limiting the use of heating tools, harsh chemicals in hair products, tight hairstyles, and excessive brushing can prevent damage to the hair shaft and minimize hair fall.

While these home remedies can aid in preventing hair loss, it's essential to remember that individual results may vary. Consultation with a healthcare professional or tricholigist is advisable, especially for persistent or severe cases of hair loss, to determine the best course of action. Combining these home remedies with professional guidance can yield more effective results in maintaining healthy, vibrant hair.

LIFESTYLE CHANGES FOR HEALTHIER HAIR

Maintaining luscious, healthy hair involves more than just external treatments. Lifestyle changes play a significant role in ensuring strong, vibrant hair that radiates health from within. Here are several lifestyle adjustments that can promote healthier hair:

1. Balanced Diet: A nutritious diet rich in vitamins, minerals, and proteins is fundamental for healthy hair. Incorporating foods like leafy greens, fruits, nuts, seeds, lean proteins, and fish provides essential nutrients like biotin, iron, zinc, and omega-3 fatty acids, crucial for hair health.

2. Hydration: Drinking an adequate amount of water daily is vital not only for overall health but also for maintaining hair hydration. Proper hydration keeps the scalp and hair follicles healthy, preventing dryness and breakage.

3. Stress Management: Stress can contribute to hair loss. Engaging in stress-reducing activities like yoga, meditation, or simply taking time for hobbies can lower stress levels, positively impacting hair health.

4. Regular Exercise: Physical activity boosts overall blood circulation, including to the scalp. This increased blood flow delivers essential nutrients to the hair follicles, promoting healthy growth.

5. Proper Hair Care Routine: Using gentle, sulfate-free shampoos and conditioners suited for your hair type, and avoiding overwashing can maintain the natural oils on the scalp. Additionally, using wide-toothed combs, minimizing heat styling, and protecting hair from sun damage can prevent breakage and damage.

6. Sufficient Sleep: Adequate sleep is essential for the body's overall rejuvenation, including hair health. During sleep, the body repairs and regenerates cells, contributing to healthier hair growth.

7. Avoiding Smoking and Excessive Alcohol: Smoking and excessive alcohol consumption can impact hair health negatively. They can restrict blood flow to the scalp, dehydrate the body, and lead to nutrient deficiencies, all of which affect hair quality.

8. Regular Trims: Getting regular trims helps eliminate split ends and prevents further damage, promoting healthier hair growth.

9. Protective Styling: Avoiding tight hairstyles and using protective styling methods, like braids or twists, can protect hair from breakage caused by tension or pulling.

Incorporating these lifestyle changes can significantly contribute to maintaining healthier hair. Consistency and patience are key, as changes may not yield immediate results. For persistent hair concerns or significant issues, consulting a healthcare professional or a dermatologist can provide tailored advice and treatments for optimal hair health.

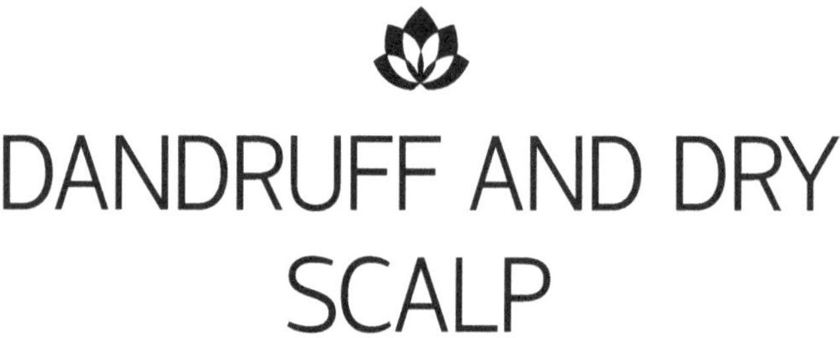

CHAPTER TWO

DANDRUFF AND DRY SCALP

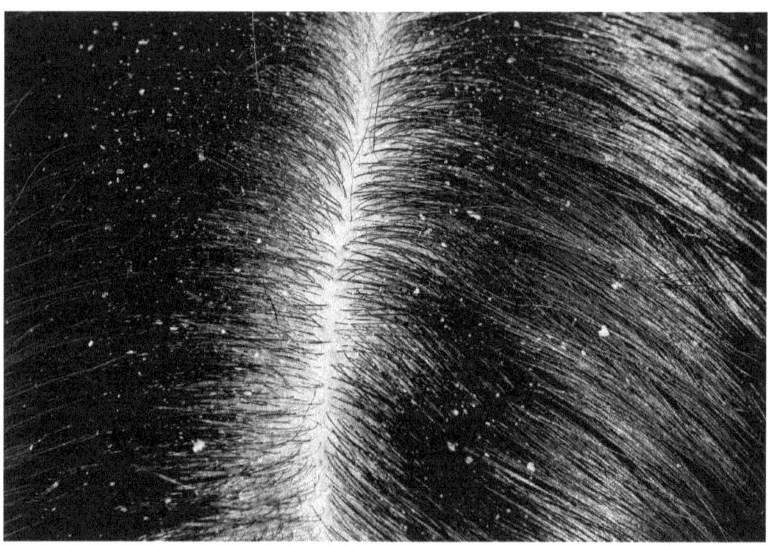

Fig. 2.1 Image showing scalp dandruff

Dandruff and dry scalp can be caused by various factors, such as dry skin, sensitivity to hair products, certain skin conditions like eczema or psoriasis, fungal infections like Malassezia, or even not shampooing enough or excessive shampooing, which can strip the scalp of its natural oils.

UNDERSTANDING THE ROOT CAUSES OF DANDRUFF AND DRY SCALP

Dandruff and dry scalp are common scalp conditions that can affect individuals of all ages, causing discomfort and sometimes embarrassment. These conditions can stem from a variety of factors, often intertwined with an individual's lifestyle, environment, and genetic predispositions.

One of the primary culprits behind dandruff and dry scalp is the natural condition of the skin. A dry scalp occurs when the skin on the scalp lacks sufficient moisture, leading to flakiness, itchiness, and irritation. This often arises due to environmental factors such as cold weather, low humidity levels, or excessive exposure to heated indoor environments. In addition, inadequate hydration or nutrition can also contribute to dry skin, impacting the scalp's health.

Another prevalent cause revolves around the proliferation of a yeast-like fungus called Malassezia. While present on everyone's scalp, an overgrowth of Malassezia can prompt irritation and trigger the accelerated shedding of skin cells. This shedding manifests as visible flakes, commonly recognized as dandruff.

Moreover, certain skin conditions, such as eczema or psoriasis, can influence the scalp's health. These conditions lead to inflammation, resulting in dryness, redness, and flaking. Individuals with these conditions might be more prone to developing dandruff or experiencing a persistently dry scalp.

Furthermore, the products one uses on their hair and scalp can significantly impact their condition. Harsh chemicals in shampoos, conditioners, or styling products can strip the scalp of its natural oils, exacerbating dryness and potentially triggering dandruff. Conversely, some individuals might be sensitive or allergic to specific ingredients in these products, causing irritation and flaking.

Additionally, irregular or excessive washing of the hair can disrupt the scalp's natural balance. Infrequent washing can lead to the buildup of oils and dead skin cells, fostering an environment conducive to dandruff. Conversely, excessive washing can strip the scalp of its natural oils, leading to dryness and flakiness.

In conclusion, dandruff and dry scalp can be attributed to a myriad of factors, including environmental conditions, fungal overgrowth, skin conditions, product usage, and hair care routines. Understanding these factors is crucial in adopting effective strategies to manage and alleviate these scalp concerns. Adjusting lifestyle habits, choosing appropriate hair products, and seeking professional advice can help individuals effectively address and manage dandruff and dry scalp, promoting a healthier scalp and more comfortable living.

Home treatments and natural remedies for dandruff and dry scalp

Here are some home treatments and natural remedies that can help alleviate dandruff and dry scalp:

Coconut Oil: Applying warm coconut oil to the scalp and leaving it on for a few hours or overnight can moisturize the scalp and help reduce dryness. It also has antibacterial properties that might help combat dandruff-causing fungus.

Tea Tree Oil: Diluted tea tree oil has antifungal properties that can help manage dandruff. Mix a few drops with a carrier oil (like coconut or olive oil) and massage it into the scalp.

Aloe Vera: Aloe vera gel has soothing properties and can alleviate scalp irritation. Apply the gel directly to the scalp and leave it for 30 minutes before rinsing.

Apple Cider Vinegar: Its acidity can help balance the pH of the scalp and reduce dandruff. Mix equal parts water and apple cider vinegar and use it as a final rinse after shampooing.

Yogurt: The probiotics in yogurt can potentially help with dandruff. Apply plain yogurt to the scalp, leave it on for about 15-20 minutes, and then rinse thoroughly.

Olive Oil: Massaging warm olive oil onto the scalp can provide moisture and alleviate dryness. Leave it on for 30-45 minutes before shampooing.

Essential Oils: Besides tea tree oil, other essential oils like lavender, rosemary, or peppermint oil, when diluted with a carrier oil, can help soothe the scalp and reduce dandruff.

Healthy Diet: Ensure your diet includes foods rich in Omega-3 fatty acids, vitamins, and minerals to support scalp health. Foods like fish, nuts, seeds, and leafy greens can be beneficial.

Reduce Stress: Stress can exacerbate scalp conditions. Practice relaxation techniques like meditation or yoga to reduce stress levels, which might improve scalp health.

Remember, individual responses to these remedies vary, so it might take some experimentation to find what works best for your scalp. It's also important to consult a Trichologist if the condition persists or worsens despite home treatments.

PROPER SCALP CARE ROUTINES FOR DANDRUFF AND DRY SCALP

Maintaining a healthy scalp is pivotal in managing and alleviating the discomfort associated with dandruff and dry scalp conditions. A well-crafted scalp care routine can significantly contribute to improving scalp health, reducing flakiness, and restoring moisture balance.

1. Choose the Right Products: Opt for gentle, pH-balanced shampoos specifically designed for dandruff or dry scalp. Look for ingredients like ketoconazole, coal tar, salicylic acid, selenium sulfide, zinc pyrithione, or tea tree oil, known for their effectiveness against dandruff-causing fungus or in soothing dryness.

2. Regular Cleansing: Wash your hair regularly, but not excessively. Frequent washing helps remove excess oil and dead skin cells, preventing buildup that can exacerbate dandruff. However, avoid daily washing as it may strip the scalp of natural oils, leading to dryness.

3. Massage Scalp: While shampooing, gently massage the scalp with fingertips to help loosen dead skin cells and improve blood circulation. Be cautious not to scratch vigorously, as this may worsen irritation.

4. Rinse Thoroughly: Ensure thorough rinsing after shampooing to eliminate any residue that might further irritate the scalp.

5. Condition Properly: Use conditioners designed for dry or sensitive scalps. Focus on applying conditioner to the hair ends, avoiding direct application to the scalp to prevent excess buildup.

6. Natural Remedies: Incorporate natural remedies like coconut oil, aloe vera, or diluted essential oils into your routine. Apply these treatments to the scalp, leaving them for a recommended duration before rinsing thoroughly.

7. Maintain Hydration: Drink plenty of water to keep your body hydrated, which in turn supports scalp moisture.

8. Diet and Nutrition: Consume a balanced diet rich in vitamins, minerals, and essential fatty acids to promote overall skin health, including the scalp. Foods like fish, nuts, seeds, fruits, and vegetables support scalp hydration and health.

9. Manage Stress: Stress management techniques like meditation, yoga, or deep breathing exercises can aid in reducing stress levels, which may positively impact scalp conditions.

Adapting these practices into a consistent scalp care routine can significantly alleviate dandruff and dry scalp issues, promoting a healthier and more comfortable scalp environment.

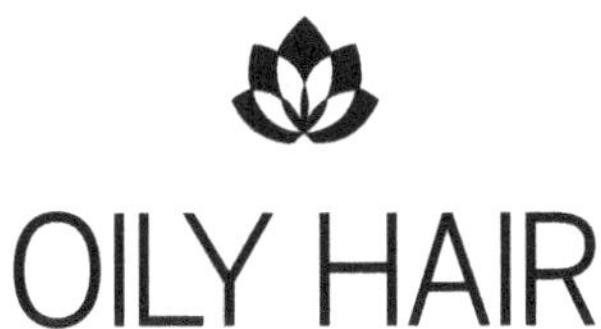

CHAPTER THREE

OILY HAIR

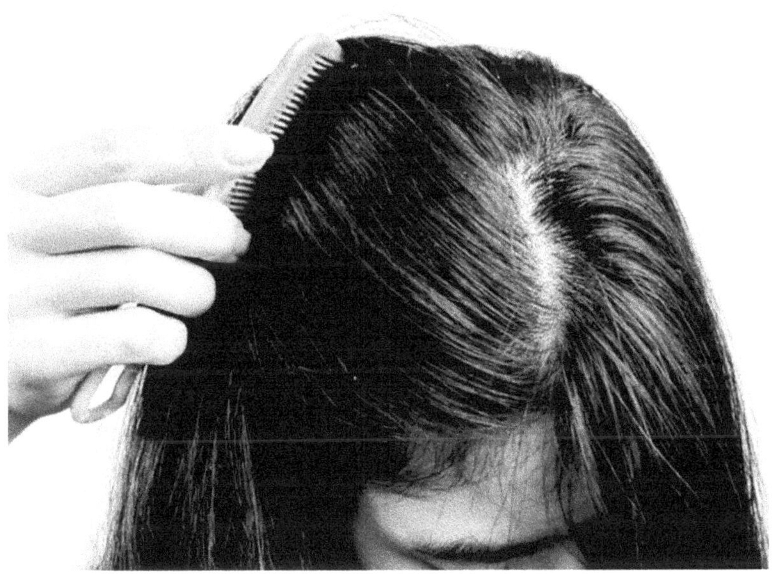

Fig. 3.1 Image showing oily scalp and hair

UNDERSTANDING OILY HAIR

Understanding oily hair is crucial for managing its care effectively. Oily hair occurs when the scalp produces excessive sebum, the natural oil that keeps hair moisturized. This overproduction can be influenced by various factors such as genetics, hormones, diet, and lifestyle.

When sebum production becomes excessive, it can make hair appear greasy and limp, often requiring more frequent washing. However, over-washing can exacerbate the issue by stripping the scalp of its natural oils, prompting the sebaceous glands to produce even more oil in response, creating a cycle.

To manage oily hair, various strategies can be employed. Using a gentle, clarifying shampoo specifically formulated for oily hair can help to cleanse the scalp without stripping it entirely. Frequent washing, though, should be balanced with not over-cleansing, as this can aggravate the condition.

Additionally, avoiding heavy or oil-based hair products can prevent further buildup. Opting for lighter, water-based products or those labeled "oil-free" can help maintain a cleaner look for longer periods. Dry shampoo can also be a handy tool to absorb excess oil between washes.

Diet and lifestyle changes can also impact sebum production. A balanced diet rich in vitamins, minerals, and omega-3 fatty acids can promote healthier hair. Furthermore, managing stress levels and avoiding excessive heat styling can contribute to healthier scalp conditions.

Understanding the unique needs of oily hair and adopting a holistic approach involving proper cleansing, suitable hair products, diet, and lifestyle adjustments can effectively manage oily hair, ensuring it looks healthy and vibrant.

You can check the oiliness of your hair by observing how quickly it becomes greasy after washing. Oily hair tends to look shiny and greasy within a day or even sooner after washing. Running your fingers through your scalp can also give you an idea – if it feels slick or oily, your hair might be on the oilier side.

HOW TO CHECK OILINESS OF SCALP AND HAIR

Visual Inspection: Look in the mirror and observe your scalp and hair. Oily hair tends to look shiny, greasy, and flat. If it appears lank and sticks together, it might be oily.

Post-Shower Observation: Notice how long it takes for your hair to appear oily after washing. If your hair looks greasy within a day or less after washing, it's likely on the oilier side.

Tactile Examination: Run your fingers along your scalp and hair. Oily hair feels slick, greasy, and might have a residue on the fingertips after touching.

Blotting Test: Use a blotting paper or tissue and press it against different parts of your scalp. Oiliness will transfer onto the paper, giving you a visual indicator of how much oil your scalp produces.

Frequency of Washing: If you find yourself needing to wash your hair frequently to get rid of the greasy appearance, it could be an indication of oily hair.

Understanding the level of oiliness can help you choose the right hair care routine and products to manage it effectively.

HOME TREATMENTS AND NATURAL REMEDIES FOR OILY HAIR

Several home treatments and natural remedies can help manage oily hair:

Apple Cider Vinegar (ACV) Rinse: Mix one part ACV with two parts water and use it as a final rinse after shampooing. It helps balance the pH of the scalp and controls oil production.

Lemon Juice: The acidity of lemon juice can help regulate oil production. Mix it with water and use it as a final rinse or add a few drops to your shampoo.

Aloe Vera: Apply aloe vera gel directly to the scalp before shampooing. It has antibacterial properties and can help control oiliness.

Tea Rinse: Brew some herbal tea (like green tea or peppermint tea), let it cool, and use it as a final rinse. These teas can help reduce excess oil.

Egg Yolk Mask: Mix egg yolk with a few drops of lemon juice and apply it to the scalp. Leave it on for 15-20 minutes before washing it off. It can help regulate oiliness while providing nourishment.

Baking Soda: It can act as a natural clarifying agent. Mix a small amount with water to form a paste, massage it into the scalp, leave for a few minutes, and rinse thoroughly.

Henna: It's not just for coloring hair; it can also help balance oil production. Use a henna mask by mixing it with water or yogurt and applying it to the scalp.

Avoid Over-Washing: Paradoxically, over-washing can stimulate more oil production. Try spacing out your washes to allow your scalp to regulate its natural oil levels.

Remember, while these remedies can help manage oily hair, it's essential to understand your hair's specific needs and consult with a Trichologist or hair care professional if you have persistent issues. Also, perform patch tests before trying new treatments to ensure you don't have any adverse reactions.

HOW TO BALANCE HAIR OIL PRODUCTION

Balancing hair oil production involves a combination of proper care, lifestyle adjustments, and using suitable products. Here's how to achieve a better balance:

Use the Right Products: Opt for gentle, sulfate-free shampoos specifically designed for oily hair. Avoid heavy conditioners or products labeled as "moisturizing" or "hydrating" for the scalp.

Regular Washing, Not Over-Washing: Wash your hair regularly to remove excess oil but avoid over-washing as it can strip the scalp of its natural oils, leading to rebound oil production.

Rinse Thoroughly: Ensure proper rinsing to remove all shampoo and conditioner residue. Residue buildup can contribute to oiliness.

Adjust Your Diet: A balanced diet rich in vitamins, minerals, and omega-3 fatty acids can positively impact hair health. Reducing processed foods and increasing intake of fruits, vegetables, and lean proteins might help balance oil production.

Stay Hydrated: Drinking plenty of water helps maintain overall skin health, including the scalp, which can impact oil production.

Use Natural Remedies: Incorporate natural remedies like apple cider vinegar rinses, tea rinses, or aloe vera applications to regulate oiliness.

Avoid Over-Styling: Limit the use of heat styling tools and hair products containing heavy oils or silicones. Heat can stimulate oil production, while heavy products can exacerbate oiliness.

Manage Stress: Stress can affect hormone levels, potentially influencing oil production. Engage in activities like meditation, exercise, or hobbies to manage stress.

Regular Scalp Massages: Gentle scalp massages can help distribute natural oils evenly and stimulate circulation, promoting a healthier scalp.

Consult a Professional: If the issue persists despite home care, consulting a dermatologist or trichologist can help identify underlying causes and provide targeted solutions.

Balancing hair oil production often involves finding the right balance between maintaining scalp health without over-stripping its natural oils. It may take some trial and error to determine the most effective routine for your hair type and lifestyle.

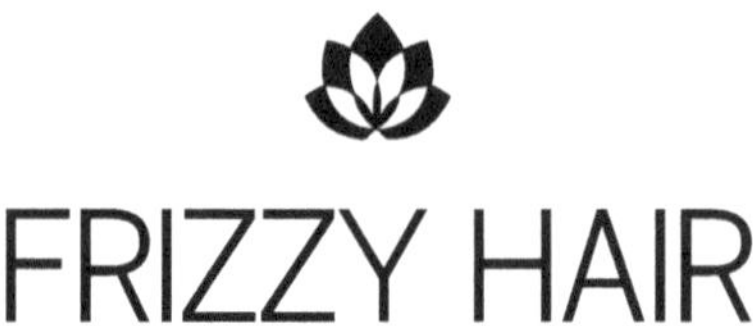

CHAPTER FOUR

FRIZZY HAIR

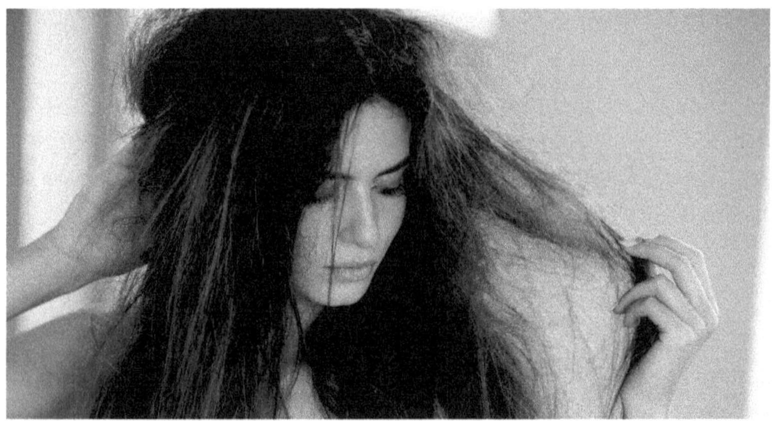

Fig. 4.1 Image showing frizzy hair

Frizzy hair refers to hair that lacks smoothness, appears dry, and forms tangles or small, wiry curls. Causes can vary, including genetics, humidity, damage from heat styling, excessive washing, lack of moisture, and certain hair products that strip natural oils or contain harsh chemicals. Frizz occurs when the hair's outer layer (cuticle) is raised, allowing moisture to enter and swell the strands, leading to the characteristic frizzy appearance.

CAUSES OF FRIZZY HAIR

Numerous causes contribute to the manifestation of frizz. Genetic predisposition plays a significant role, as hair type and texture are hereditary. For instance, individuals with naturally curly or wavy hair are more prone to frizz due to the hair's structure and tendency to trap moisture.

Environmental factors, such as humidity, play a pivotal role in exacerbating frizz. In high-humidity conditions, the hair's outer layer, known as the cuticle, absorbs moisture from the atmosphere, causing the strands to swell. This absorption leads to the raised cuticle, creating a frizzy appearance as the hair attempts to find space for the increased volume.

Moreover, damage caused by heat styling tools like flat irons, curling wands, or blow dryers contributes significantly to frizz. Excessive heat strips the hair of its natural moisture, weakening the cuticle and making it more susceptible to environmental influences.

Frequent washing with harsh shampoos or overuse of styling products containing alcohol or sulfates can also strip the hair of its natural oils, leaving it dry and prone to frizz. Additionally, certain hair treatments, chemical processes, and even brushing hair aggressively when wet can contribute to frizz by causing damage to the hair's structure.

Effective management of frizzy hair involves various strategies. Hydration is crucial, achieved through the use of moisturizing shampoos, conditioners, and leave-in treatments that help nourish and replenish lost moisture. Incorporating regular deep conditioning and oil treatments can also aid in restoring the hair's health and manageability.

Protective styling, such as braids or buns, can shield the hair from environmental factors, reducing exposure to humidity. Limiting heat styling and opting for heat protectant products can mitigate damage, preserving the hair's natural moisture and minimizing frizz.

In conclusion, the definition and causes of frizzy hair are multifaceted, encompassing genetic predisposition, environmental influences like humidity, damage from heat styling, excessive washing, and the use of harsh hair products. Effective management involves a combination of hydration, protection, and minimizing practices that strip the hair of its natural oils, ultimately restoring and maintaining the hair's health and manageability.

DIY TREATMENTS FOR MANAGING FRIZZINESS OF HAIR

Here are a few DIY treatments that can help manage frizzy hair:

Coconut Oil Mask: Apply warm coconut oil generously to your hair, focusing on the ends. Leave it on for 30 minutes to an hour before shampooing. Coconut oil deeply moisturizes and nourishes the hair, reducing frizz.

Apple Cider Vinegar Rinse: Mix equal parts of water and apple cider vinegar. After shampooing, pour the mixture over your hair, let it sit for a few minutes, then rinse. This helps balance the hair's pH levels, sealing the cuticles and reducing frizz.

Banana and Avocado Hair Mask: Blend a ripe banana and half an avocado. Apply this mixture to damp hair and leave it on for 20-30 minutes before rinsing. Both fruits contain natural oils and vitamins that can hydrate and smoothen frizzy hair.

Aloe Vera Gel Treatment: Apply aloe vera gel directly to damp hair, focusing on the frizzy areas. Leave it on for 20-30 minutes before rinsing. Aloe vera helps in moisturizing and taming frizz.

Honey and Olive Oil Hair Mask: Mix equal parts honey and olive oil, then apply it to damp hair. Leave it on for 20-30 minutes before rinsing thoroughly. The combination of honey's humectant properties and olive oil's moisturizing effects can help manage frizz.

Remember, consistency is key with these treatments. While they might not completely eliminate frizz, regular use can significantly improve the condition and manageability of frizzy hair.

TIPS FOR PREVENTING FRIZZY HAIR

Here are some effective tips to help prevent frizzy hair:

Use a Moisturizing Shampoo and Conditioner: Look for products specifically designed to hydrate and nourish the hair. Avoid shampoos containing sulfates, as they can strip the hair of its natural oils, contributing to frizz.

Limit Washing and Use Lukewarm Water: Wash your hair less frequently to retain natural oils. When washing, use lukewarm water instead of hot water, which can dry out the hair and increase frizz.

Apply a Leave-In Conditioner or Serum: After washing your hair, apply a leave-in conditioner or serum to lock in moisture and keep the hair hydrated throughout the day. Focus on the ends and areas prone to frizz.

Avoid Heat Styling: Reduce the use of heat styling tools like flat irons, curling wands, and blow dryers. If you must use them, apply a heat protectant spray or serum beforehand to minimize damage.

Pat Dry, Don't Rub: After washing your hair, gently pat it dry with a microfiber towel or an old cotton t-shirt. Avoid rubbing vigorously, as this can roughen up the hair cuticle and lead to frizz.

Use a Wide-Tooth Comb or a Detangling Brush: When brushing your hair, use a wide-tooth comb or a brush specifically designed for detangling to minimize breakage and prevent frizz.

Protect Your Hair From Humidity: In high-humidity environments, protect your hair by using anti-humidity hair products or styling creams to create a barrier against moisture absorption.

Trim Regularly: Regular trims help get rid of split ends, which can contribute to frizz. Aim for a trim every 6-8 weeks to maintain healthy ends.

Sleep on Silk or Satin Pillowcases: These materials create less friction, reducing the likelihood of frizz compared to cotton pillowcases. They also help retain moisture in the hair.

Consider Protective Hairstyles: Braids, buns, or other protective hairstyles can shield your hair from environmental factors and minimize exposure to humidity, reducing frizz.

Combining these preventive measures can significantly help in managing and reducing frizz, keeping your hair healthier and more manageable in the long run.

CHAPTER FIVE

SPLIT ENDS AND HAIR BREAKAGE

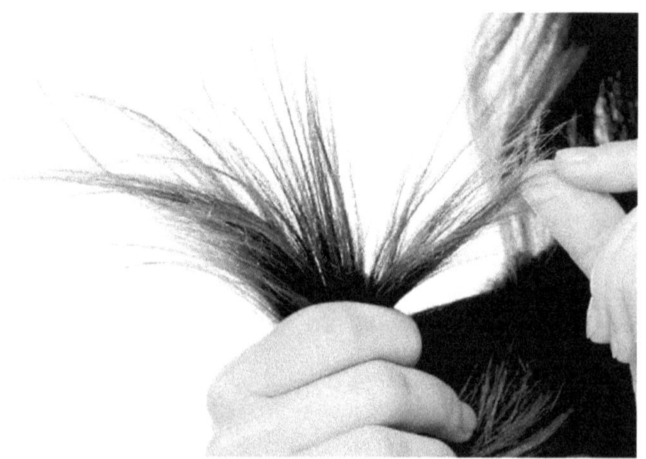

Fig. 5.1 Image showing split ends

Split ends refer to the splitting or fraying of the hair shaft, typically occurring at the tips of the hair. This happens when the protective outer layer of the hair cuticle is damaged or wears away, resulting in the hair splitting into two or more strands.

CAUSES OF SPLIT ENDS IN HAIR

Hair is an integral part of our identity, but split ends can often plague its health and appearance. These split ends, medically termed as "trichoptilosis," occur when the hair shaft splits or frays, resulting in a frazzled appearance. Several factors contribute to this common hair woe.

1. Excessive Heat Styling: Regular use of heated styling tools such as straighteners, curling irons, or blow dryers can weaken the hair shaft, leading to dehydration and breakage, thereby causing split ends.

2. Harsh Chemicals: Chemical treatments like bleaching, perming, or coloring can strip the hair of its natural oils and weaken its structure, making it prone to splitting.

3. Over-washing and Harsh Products: Frequent washing or using harsh shampoos and conditioners can strip the hair of its natural oils, leaving it dry and vulnerable to breakage.

4. Environmental Factors: Exposure to environmental elements like UV rays, pollution, wind, and extreme temperatures can damage the hair cuticle, causing split ends.

5. Rough Handling: Brushing or combing hair too vigorously, especially when wet, can cause stress on the strands, leading to breakage and split ends.

6. Poor Nutrition: A lack of essential nutrients like vitamins, minerals, and proteins in one's diet can affect hair health, making it more prone to damage and split ends.

7. Genetic Predisposition: Some individuals naturally have hair that is more prone to splitting due to genetic factors or inherent hair structure.

Preventing split ends involves a combination of proper hair care practices and lifestyle adjustments. Trim hair regularly to remove existing split ends and prevent them from traveling up the hair shaft. Use heat protectants before styling with hot tools, opt for gentle hair care products suitable for your hair type, minimize chemical treatments, protect hair from environmental stressors, and maintain a balanced diet to support healthy hair growth.

In conclusion, split ends in hair are a common issue caused by a variety of factors, ranging from our daily hair care routines to environmental influences and genetic predispositions. By adopting gentle hair care practices and making conscious lifestyle choices, one can significantly reduce the occurrence of split ends and promote overall hair health.

HOME REMEDIES FOR REPAIRING AND PREVENTING DAMAGE

Certainly! Here are some home remedies to repair and prevent hair damage:

1. Coconut Oil: Apply warm coconut oil to your hair and scalp, leaving it on for a few hours or overnight before washing. This helps moisturize and protect hair from damage.

2. Egg Mask: Create a mask using eggs, mixing them with olive oil and honey. Apply this to your hair, leaving it for about 20 minutes before rinsing with cool water. Eggs contain proteins that can strengthen hair.

3. Avocado Mask: Mash a ripe avocado and combine it with coconut oil or honey. Apply this mask to your hair, leaving it on for 20-30 minutes before rinsing. Avocado provides nourishment to damaged hair.

4. Aloe Vera: Apply aloe vera gel directly to the scalp to soothe and moisturize. It helps in repairing damaged cells on the scalp.

5. Apple Cider Vinegar Rinse: Mix apple cider vinegar with water and use it as a final rinse after shampooing. It helps restore the pH balance of the scalp and adds shine to hair.

Incorporating these remedies into your routine can help repair damage and prevent further harm to your hair, promoting its overall health and strength.

BEST PRACTICES FOR REDUCING SPLIT ENDS

Reducing split ends involves adopting several practices to maintain healthier hair:

1. Regular Trims: Get regular haircuts every 6-8 weeks to remove split ends and prevent them from traveling up the hair shaft.

2. Gentle Handling: Avoid aggressive brushing, especially when hair is wet. Use a wide-tooth comb or a brush designed for detangling to minimize breakage.

3. Minimize Heat Styling: Limit the use of heat styling tools or use them on lower heat settings. Always use a heat protectant before styling.

4. Avoid Harsh Chemicals: Minimize exposure to harsh chemical treatments like bleaching, perming, and excessive coloring.

5. Moisturize and Condition: Use a hydrating conditioner after every wash to nourish and protect your hair. Consider using leave-in conditioners or masks for added moisture.

6. Protect from Environmental Stress: Wear hats or use protective products when exposed to sun, wind, or extreme temperatures to shield hair from environmental damage.

7. Proper Washing Techniques: Wash hair with lukewarm water instead of hot water, and avoid over-washing, as it can strip the hair of natural oils.

8. Diet and Hydration: Maintain a balanced diet rich in proteins, vitamins (especially A, C, and E), and minerals like zinc and iron. Drink plenty of water to keep your body and hair hydrated.

9. Silk or Satin Pillowcases: Switching to silk or satin pillowcases can reduce friction, preventing breakage and split ends while you sleep.

10. Protective Hairstyles: Opt for hairstyles that protect the ends, like buns or braids, to minimize exposure to friction and environmental damage.

Incorporating these practices into your hair care routine can significantly reduce split ends, keeping your hair healthier and more manageable.

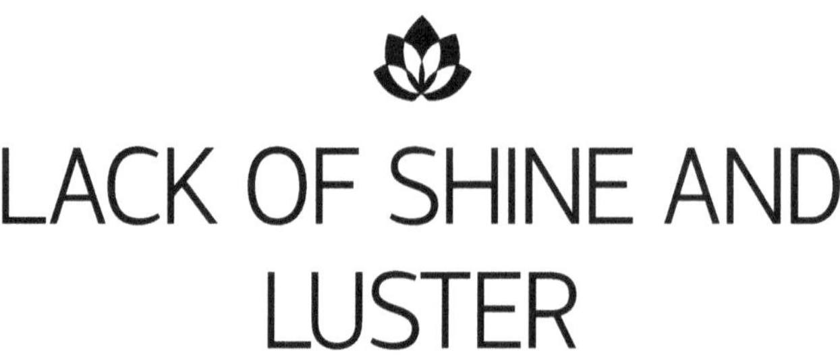

LACK OF SHINE AND LUSTER

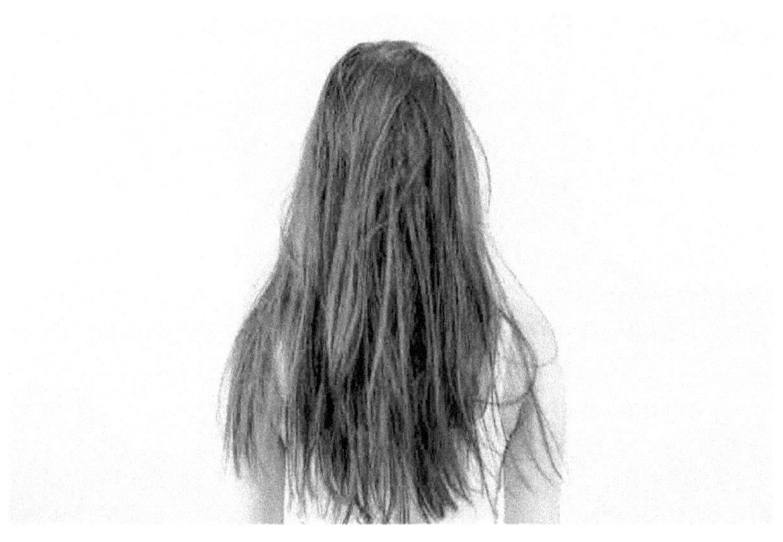

Fig. 6.1 Image showing lusterless hair

Dull hair refers to hair that lacks shine, looks lifeless, and feels rough or dry. It often occurs due to various factors like damage from styling, exposure to harsh chemicals, excessive washing, or lack of proper nutrients.

CAUSES OF DULL HAIR

Hair, often considered a crowning glory, loses its luster due to multiple factors. Dullness in hair can be attributed to various causes, ranging from environmental factors to personal habits and health issues.

Over-Styling: Excessive use of heat styling tools like straighteners, curlers, or blow dryers can strip the hair of its natural oils, leading to a lack of shine and vitality.

Chemical Treatments: Regular exposure to harsh chemicals from coloring, perming, or chemical straightening damages the hair cuticle, making it prone to dryness and lack of shine.

Environmental Factors: Pollution, sun exposure, and harsh weather conditions can contribute to the accumulation of dirt, pollutants, and UV damage on the hair, causing it to appear dull and lifeless.

Poor Hair Care Habits: Infrequent washing or using harsh shampoos that contain sulfates can strip the hair of its natural oils, making it look dull and lackluster.

Nutritional Deficiencies: Inadequate intake of essential nutrients like vitamins, minerals, and proteins can affect hair health. Deficiencies in vitamins such as Biotin, Vitamin E, and Omega-3 fatty acids can result in dry, lackluster hair.

Stress and Lifestyle Factors: Stress, lack of sleep, and an unhealthy lifestyle can impact overall health, leading to poor hair quality and dullness.

Genetic Predisposition: Some individuals may inherently have hair that tends towards dullness due to genetic factors, making it harder to maintain shine without proper care.

Aging: As individuals age, the natural oil production in the scalp decreases, causing hair to become drier and lose its natural shine.

Preventing or mitigating dullness in hair involves adopting healthy hair care practices. Regular conditioning, minimizing heat exposure, protecting hair from environmental damage, eating a balanced diet rich in essential nutrients, and proper hydration all contribute to maintaining hair's shine and vitality.

In conclusion, various factors, from external environmental influences to internal health and lifestyle choices, play a crucial role in the appearance and health of our hair. Understanding these causes helps in adopting suitable hair care routines to prevent or address dullness, ensuring that our hair remains a reflection of health and vitality.

DIY TREATMENTS FOR RESTORING HAIR SHINE

Dull, lackluster hair can often be rejuvenated and brought back to life through simple do-it-yourself treatments using natural ingredients. These remedies aim to nourish and hydrate the hair, restoring its natural shine and vitality.

Coconut Oil Mask: Coconut oil is rich in fatty acids that penetrate the hair shaft, providing deep hydration and shine. Apply warm coconut oil to damp hair, focusing on the ends, and leave it on for at least 30 minutes or overnight before washing it out.

Apple Cider Vinegar Rinse: An apple cider vinegar rinse helps to restore the pH balance of the scalp, remove buildup, and seal the hair cuticles, resulting in shinier, smoother hair. Mix equal parts of water and apple cider vinegar, use it as a final rinse after shampooing, then rinse with water.

Avocado Hair Mask: Avocado is packed with vitamins, essential fatty acids, and minerals that deeply moisturize and add shine to hair. Mash a ripe avocado and mix it with a tablespoon of olive oil or honey. Apply this mask to clean, damp hair, leave it for 20-30 minutes, then rinse thoroughly.

Egg Yolk Treatment: Egg yolks are rich in proteins and fats, making them an excellent natural conditioner. Beat 1-2 egg yolks and apply the mixture to damp hair, leave it on for 20 minutes, then rinse with cool water. This treatment helps add shine and strength to dull hair.

Honey and Yogurt Mask: Honey is a humectant that attracts moisture, while yogurt contains lactic acid that cleanses and adds shine. Mix equal parts of honey and plain yogurt, apply it to clean, damp hair, leave it on for 20-30 minutes, then rinse thoroughly.

Aloe Vera Gel Treatment: Aloe vera contains enzymes that promote healthy hair growth and restore shine. Apply fresh aloe vera gel directly to the scalp and hair, leave it on for 30 minutes, then rinse it out.

Regularly incorporating these DIY treatments into a hair care routine can help nourish and revitalize dull hair, bringing back its natural shine and luster without resorting to harsh chemicals or expensive products.

In conclusion, nature offers an array of potent ingredients that can be used to restore hair shine and health. These DIY treatments not only rejuvenate dull hair but also promote overall hair health, leaving you with shiny, vibrant locks.

TIPS FOR MAINTAINING HAIR'S NATURAL LUSTER

Maintaining your hair's natural luster involves a combination of proper care and healthy habits. Here are some tips to help maintain that shine:

Regular Conditioning: Use a quality conditioner after shampooing to hydrate and smooth the hair cuticle, promoting shine and manageability. Consider deep conditioning treatments occasionally for extra nourishment.

Avoid Over-Shampooing: Washing hair too frequently can strip away natural oils, leading to dryness and dullness. Opt for a gentle shampoo and wash your hair as needed, not excessively.

Cool Water Rinse: Finish your shower with a cool water rinse. Cold water helps seal the hair cuticles, making your hair look smoother and shinier.

Protect from Heat: Minimize heat exposure from styling tools. If you must use heat, apply a heat protectant and use the lowest temperature setting possible.

Trim Regularly: Regular trims prevent split ends, which can make hair appear frizzy and dull. Aim for a trim every 6-8 weeks to maintain healthy ends.

Balanced Diet: Eat a nutrient-rich diet with plenty of protein, vitamins (especially Biotin, Vitamin E, and Omega-3 fatty acids), and minerals to support healthy hair growth and shine.

Hydration: Stay hydrated! Drinking enough water is crucial for overall hair health and maintaining its natural shine.

Protect from Environmental Damage: Wear hats or use products with UV protection to shield your hair from sun damage and environmental pollutants.

Avoid Harsh Chemicals: Limit chemical treatments and use gentle, sulfate-free products to prevent damage to the hair shaft.

Use Natural Remedies: Incorporate natural remedies like coconut oil, aloe vera, or avocado into your hair care routine to nourish and restore shine.

Consistency with these practices will help maintain your hair's natural luster, keeping it healthy, shiny, and vibrant.

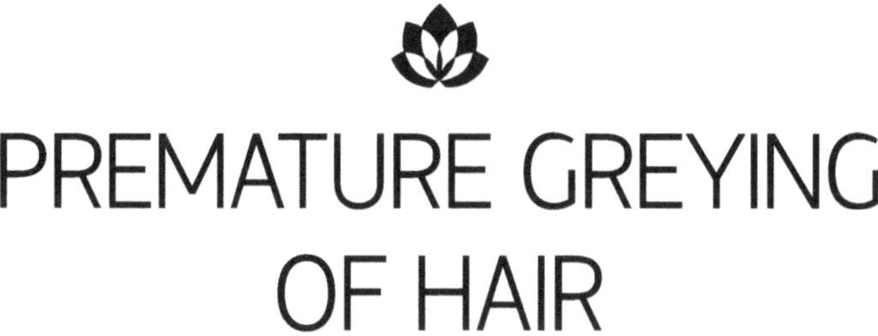

CHAPTER SEVEN

PREMATURE GREYING OF HAIR

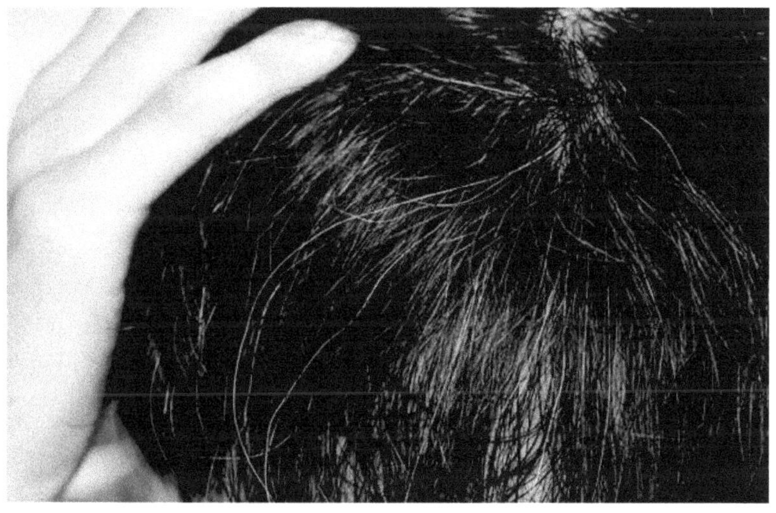

Fig. 7.1 Image showing graying of hair in a teen age boy

Premature graying refers to the early onset of gray or white hair before the age at which it is typically expected, usually before the mid-20s for Caucasians and mid-30s for Asians.

CAUSES OF PREMATURE GREYING

Premature graying of hair can occur due to a variety of reasons:

Genetics: Family history and genetic predisposition play a significant role. If your parents or grandparents experienced premature graying, there's a higher chance you might too.

Deficiency in Melanin Production: Melanin gives hair its color. Any disruption or reduction in melanin production due to various factors can lead to premature graying.

Vitamin and Mineral Deficiencies: Deficiencies in vitamins like B12, D, E, and minerals such as iron, copper, and zinc can affect melanin production, accelerating graying.

Health Conditions: Certain health conditions like thyroid disorders, vitiligo, anemia, and autoimmune diseases can impact melanin production and contribute to premature graying.

Stress: Chronic stress can affect the body in numerous ways, including hair health. It might speed up the graying process by disrupting melanin production.

Environmental Factors: Exposure to pollutants, toxins, and chemicals, as well as excessive exposure to the sun's UV radiation, can damage hair and contribute to premature graying.

Lifestyle Choices: Smoking, an unhealthy diet lacking essential nutrients, and poor lifestyle habits can also hasten premature graying.

Understanding these various causes can help in making lifestyle changes or seeking appropriate medical advice to manage or slow down premature graying.

HOME REMEDIES TO TREAT PREMATURE GREYING

Several home remedies are believed to help manage premature graying, although scientific evidence supporting their effectiveness might be limited.

Amla (Indian Gooseberry): Amla is rich in antioxidants and vitamin C, which may help with hair health. Consuming amla juice or applying amla oil to the scalp is thought to be beneficial.

Curry Leaves: Curry leaves are believed to contain nutrients that can help restore pigment to the hair. Boiling curry leaves in coconut oil and applying this oil to the hair can be a popular remedy.

Coconut Oil and Lemon Juice: A mixture of coconut oil and lemon juice is thought to nourish the scalp and potentially slow down premature graying. Massaging this mixture onto the scalp could be beneficial.

Onion Juice: Onion juice contains catalase, an enzyme that may help in reversing graying. Applying onion juice to the scalp is a traditional remedy.

Henna: Henna is a natural dye that can cover gray hair. However, it might provide temporary results and may not suit everyone.

Remember, while these remedies are often used and passed down through generations, their effectiveness might vary from person to person. It's essential to consult a healthcare professional or a Trichologist before extensively relying on home remedies, especially if you have underlying health conditions or allergies.

TIPS FOR PREVENTING PREMATURE GREYING

Here are some tips that might help prevent premature graying:

Healthy Diet: Consume a balanced diet rich in vitamins, minerals, and antioxidants. Foods like leafy greens, nuts, seeds, and fruits provide essential nutrients for hair health.

Manage Stress: Stress management techniques such as meditation, exercise, or mindfulness can potentially slow down premature graying.

Avoid Smoking: Smoking is linked to premature aging, including premature graying. Quitting smoking might help slow down the graying process.

Good Hair Care: Use mild shampoos and conditioners suitable for your hair type. Avoid excessive heat styling and harsh chemical treatments that can damage hair.

Adequate Sleep: Ensure you get enough quality sleep as it plays a vital role in overall health, including hair health.

Protect from Environmental Factors: Shield your hair from excessive sun exposure, pollutants, and chemicals. Wearing hats or scarves can help protect your hair from environmental damage.

Regular Scalp Massages: Massaging the scalp can improve blood circulation to the hair follicles, promoting hair health.

While these tips may support overall hair health, it's important to note that genetics and other uncontrollable factors might still influence premature graying.

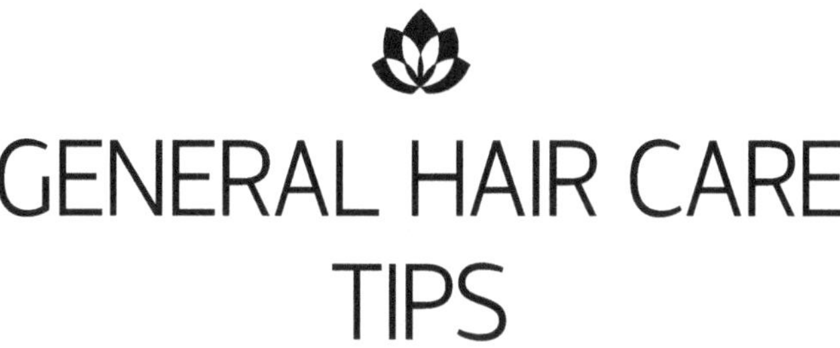

CHAPTER EIGHT

GENERAL HAIR CARE TIPS

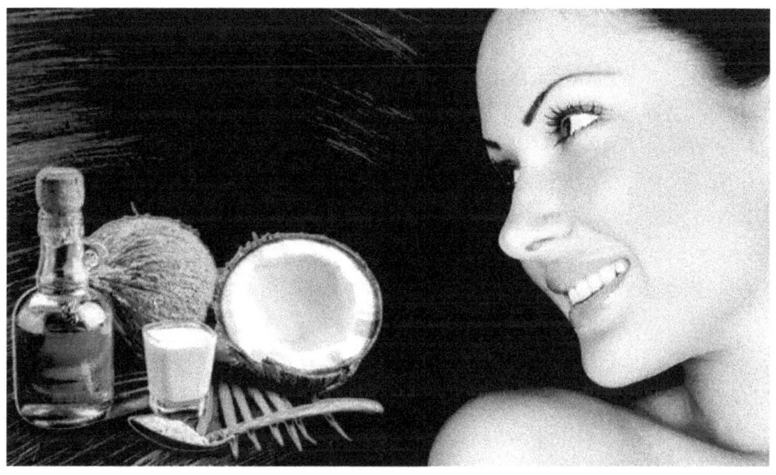

Fig.8.1 Happy female with healthy hair

BEST PRACTICES FOR HEALTHY HAIR

Maintaining healthy hair involves a blend of care, lifestyle choices, and grooming habits. The key practices for fostering healthy hair include:

1. Proper Nutrition: A balanced diet rich in proteins, vitamins (especially A, C, D, and E), minerals (like iron and zinc), and omega-3 fatty acids supports hair health.

2. Gentle Washing: Use a mild shampoo suited to your hair type and wash it 2-3 times a week. Overwashing can strip the hair of its natural oils, leading to dryness.

3. Condition Regularly: Apply conditioner after shampooing to restore moisture, reduce tangles, and maintain hair strength.

4. Limit Heat Styling: Excessive heat from blow dryers, curling irons, and straighteners damages the hair. Use heat protectants and try air-drying whenever possible.

5. Protective Hairstyles: Minimize strain on hair by avoiding tight hairstyles that pull on the scalp. Opt for looser styles to prevent breakage and hair loss.

6. Regular Trims: Trimming split ends every 6-8 weeks prevents them from traveling up the hair shaft, keeping your hair healthy and manageable.

7. Scalp Care: A healthy scalp fosters healthy hair growth. Keep your scalp clean and massage it regularly to stimulate blood flow.

8. Avoid Harsh Chemicals: Limit the use of harsh chemical treatments like perms, bleaching, and coloring. If used, ensure proper care and conditioning thereafter.

9. Protect from Environmental Damage: Shield your hair from the sun, wind, and pollutants by using hats or scarves.

10. Hydration: Drink plenty of water to keep your body—and consequently, your hair—hydrated.

11. Stress Management: Stress negatively impacts hair health. Incorporate stress-reducing activities into your routine to promote overall well-being, benefiting your hair health too.

Adopting these practices consistently forms the foundation for healthy, vibrant hair. It's essential to understand your hair's unique needs and adjust routines accordingly for optimal care.

NUTRITION AND DIET FOR GOOD HAIR HEALTH

A well-rounded diet contributes significantly to healthy hair. Incorporating these nutrients can promote optimal hair health:

1. Protein: Hair is primarily made of protein, so include sources like lean meats, fish, eggs, dairy, legumes, and nuts to support hair growth.

2. Omega-3 Fatty Acids: Found in fish, flaxseeds, chia seeds, and walnuts, these fatty acids nourish the scalp and support hair hydration.

3. Vitamins:

Vitamin A: Encourages healthy production of sebum, the scalp's natural oil. Carrots, sweet potatoes, and spinach are rich sources.

Vitamin C: Assists in collagen production, crucial for hair structure. Citrus fruits, berries, and peppers are excellent sources.

Vitamin D: Promotes hair follicle health. Sunlight exposure, fortified foods, and supplements help.

Vitamin E: Enhances blood circulation to the scalp. Almonds, sunflower seeds, and spinach contain high levels.

4. Iron: Anemia can cause hair loss, so ensure you have iron-rich foods like red meat, spinach, lentils, and fortified cereals.

5. Zinc: Supports hair growth and repair. Consume oysters, nuts, seeds, and whole grains for adequate zinc intake.

6. Biotin: Known as B7, it's crucial for hair strength and growth. Eggs, nuts, whole grains, and bananas are good sources.

7. Water: Hydration is key for healthy hair growth. Drink enough water to maintain overall hydration.

A balanced diet that includes these nutrients not only supports hair health but also benefits overall wellness. Consulting a healthcare professional or a registered dietitian can provide personalized guidance for optimal nutritional intake.

STYLING TIPS AND DAMAGING HABITS FOR HAIR

Here are some insights into both styling tips and damaging habits that affect hair health:

Styling Tips for Healthy Hair:

Use Heat Protectants: Before using heat styling tools, apply a protectant to minimize damage caused by high temperatures.

Air Dry Whenever Possible: Limit heat exposure by allowing your hair to air dry instead of using blow dryers.

Choose Gentle Accessories: Use hair ties, clips, and accessories that are gentle on the hair to avoid breakage.

Regular Trimming: Schedule regular trims to prevent split ends from traveling up the hair shaft, keeping your hair healthy.

Protect from the Sun: Shield your hair from UV damage by wearing hats or using products with UV protection.

Damaging Habits to Avoid:

Overuse of Heat Styling: Excessive use of straighteners, curling irons, or blow dryers can cause damage, leading to dryness and breakage.

Tight Hairstyles: Constantly styling hair in tight ponytails, braids, or buns can cause tension on the hair follicles, resulting in breakage and hair loss.

Chemical Overprocessing: Frequent coloring, perming, or chemical straightening can weaken the hair, making it prone to damage and breakage.

Skipping Heat Protectants: Neglecting to use heat protectants before using styling tools increases the risk of heat damage.

Rough Towel Drying: Vigorously rubbing wet hair with a towel can cause friction and breakage. Instead, gently pat or squeeze excess water out of the hair.

Over-washing: Washing hair too frequently strips it of natural oils, leading to dryness and potential damage.

BALANCING STYLING AND HEALTHY HAIR PRACTICES

Understanding your hair type and its specific needs is crucial in maintaining a balance between styling and preserving hair health. Implementing protective measures, limiting damaging habits, and adopting a gentle hair care routine contribute to overall hair health and vitality.

Consistency in good hair care practices, coupled with occasional pampering and attention to potential damaging habits, is key to maintaining healthy, lustrous hair.

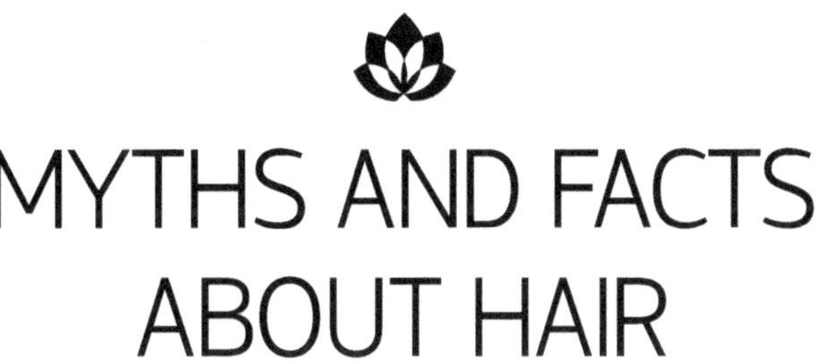

CHAPTER NINE

MYTHS AND FACTS ABOUT HAIR

HAIR MYTHS

1. CUTTING YOUR HAIR MAKES IT GROW FASTER

One of the most enduring myths about hair is that cutting it will make it grow faster. In reality, hair growth occurs at the scalp, not at the tips. Hair growth is primarily influenced by genetics, diet, and overall health. Trimming the ends of your hair can prevent split ends and breakage, which may give the illusion of faster growth, but it doesn't affect the rate at which hair grows from the roots.

1. FREQUENT SHAMPOOING CAUSES HAIR LOSS

Some individuals avoid frequent shampooing out of fear that it will lead to hair loss. In reality, washing your hair regularly is essential for maintaining a healthy scalp and hair. Overuse of harsh shampoos or excessive heat styling can damage hair, but simply washing it regularly is not a cause of hair loss. In fact, keeping your scalp clean can promote hair health.

3. PLUCKING ONE GRAY HAIR CAUSES MORE TO GROW

A widespread myth is that plucking a single gray hair will lead to the growth of multiple gray hairs in its place. This notion is entirely false. Plucking a gray hair only removes that specific hair, and it will not influence the color of surrounding hair. However, it's best to avoid excessive plucking, as it can damage the hair follicle and lead to hair loss.

4. HAIR GROWS THICKER AND DARKER AFTER SHAVING

Many people believe that shaving or cutting hair will make it grow back thicker and darker. This is a persistent myth. Shaving or cutting hair does not alter its texture or color. What may give this impression is the fact that newly grown hair has a blunt edge, which can appear thicker than hair that has naturally tapered ends.

5. HAIR GROWS CONTINUOUSLY THROUGHOUT LIFE

Contrary to popular belief, hair doesn't grow continuously. It goes through growth cycles that include growth (anagen), rest (telogen), and shedding phases. Each hair follicle has its own cycle, and not all hairs are in the same phase at the same time.

6. BRUSHING HAIR 100 STROKES A DAY MAKES IT HEALTHIER

Excessive brushing can actually damage hair by causing breakage and stress on the strands. Gentle brushing to detangle and distribute natural oils is beneficial, but 100 strokes a day is unnecessary and may lead to more harm than good.

7. HAIR CAN "BREATHE" THROUGH THE SCALP

Hair isn't a living structure, so it doesn't "breathe" in the way our lungs do. It receives nutrients and oxygen from lood vessels in the scalp. However, a clean and healthy scalp can support optimal hair growth.

8. HAIR LOSS IS ONLY A MEN'S ISSUE

While male pattern baldness is more common and noticeable, women can also experience hair loss due to various factors such as genetics, hormonal changes, stress, and medical conditions.

9. NATURAL OILS ARE ALWAYS GOOD FOR HAIR

While some natural oils like coconut or argan oil can be beneficial for hair, not all oils are suitable for all hair types. Using the wrong oil can lead to greasiness or buildup. It's essential to choose products that suit your hair's specific needs.

10. WEARING HATS CAUSES BALDNESS

Wearing hats, even regularly, does not lead to baldness. Hair loss occurs due to genetic, hormonal, or health factors, not from wearing hats. However, hats that are very tight and cause constant friction might contribute to hair breakage.

11. HAIR CAN TURN WHITE OVERNIGHT FROM SHOCK

It's a common myth that extreme shock or fear can turn hair white overnight. While stress can contribute to hair graying over time, the process is gradual and not caused by a single traumatic event.

12. WASHING HAIR WITH BEER MAKES IT SHINY

Beer contains certain proteins and nutrients that might temporarily add shine to hair due to their coating properties. However, this effect is short-lived and doesn't provide lasting benefits. It's not a recommended hair care practice.

13. CUTTING HAIR DURING A FULL MOON MAKES IT GROW FASTER

This myth is based on superstition and has no scientific basis. Hair growth is primarily influenced by genetics and other internal factors, not the lunar cycle.

14. SHAVING HAIR OFF WILL MAKE IT GROW BACK THICKER

Shaving any part of your body, including the head, does not change the thickness or texture of hair. The hair that grows back after shaving is the same as before.

15. BALDNESS COMES FROM YOUR MOTHER'S SIDE OF THE FAMILY

While genetics play a significant role in hair loss, it's not solely determined by your mother's side. Baldness genes can be inherited from both parents.

16. YOU LOSE MOST OF YOUR BODY HEAT THROUGH YOUR HEAD

The myth that you lose most of your body heat through your head is not entirely accurate. Heat loss depends on the surface area exposed to cold air. While it's essential to keep your head warm in cold weather, it's not the only source of heat loss.

17. BRUSHING HAIR 100 STROKES A DAY STIMULATES HAIR GROWTH

This myth suggests that brushing your hair vigorously 100 times a day will promote faster hair growth. In reality, excessive brushing can lead to hair breakage and damage. Gentle brushing to detangle and distribute natural oils is sufficient.

18. HAIR COLOR CAN INDICATE PERSONALITY TRAITS

Some people believe that hair color is linked to personality traits, such as blondes being perceived as less intelligent or brunettes as more serious. These stereotypes have no scientific basis and should not be used to judge individuals.

19. HENNA IS SAFE FOR ALL HAIR TYPES

While henna is a natural dye derived from the henna plant, it can interact with other hair treatments or chemicals. It's not always safe for all hair types, especially if you have previously used chemical dyes or treatments. A patch test is recommended before full application.

20. WASHING HAIR LESS OFTEN MAKES IT LESS GREASY

Some people believe that if they wash their hair less frequently, it will become less greasy over time. In reality, washing hair regularly helps remove excess oil and maintain scalp health. Washing less often may cause the scalp to produce more oil in response.

21. HAIR LOSS IS ONLY A SIGN OF AGING

Hair loss can occur at any age and may result from various factors, including genetics, hormonal changes, medical conditions, and stress. It's not solely a sign of aging, and young people can experience hair loss too.

22. HAIR CAN BE PERMANENTLY STRAIGHTENED OR CURLED WITHOUT CHEMICALS

While there are treatments like keratin straightening and perms that can temporarily change the hair's texture, these effects are not permanent. Over time, your natural hair texture will return.

23. HONEY CAN LIGHTEN HAIR COLOR NATURALLY

Some people believe that applying honey to their hair and sitting in the sun will naturally lighten their hair color. While honey may slightly lighten hair due to its natural hydrogen peroxide content, the effect is subtle and may not work for everyone.

Conclusion: Understanding these hair myths and distinguishing them from facts can help individuals make informed choices about their hair care routines and dispel common misconceptions that may influence their decisions. Healthy hair care practices are essential for maintaining vibrant and beautiful hair.

HAIR FACTS

1. Hair is made up of a protein called keratin.The average person has about 100,000 to 150,000 hair follicles on their scalp.
2. Hair growth occurs in cycles, with each hair strand having a growth phase, rest phase, and shedding phase.
3. Hair grows at an average rate of about half an inch (1.25 cm) per month.
4. The color of your hair is determined by the amount and type of melanin in your hair follicles.
5. There are two main types of melanin: eumelanin (responsible for brown and black hair) and pheomelanin (responsible for red and blonde hair).
6. Gray hair occurs when melanin production decreases with age.
7. Hair can be straight, wavy, or curly, depending on the shape of the hair follicle.
8. On average, people lose 50 to 100 hairs from their scalp each day.
9. Hair is composed of three layers: the medulla, cortex, and cuticle.
10. The medulla is the innermost layer of hair and is often absent in fine hair.

11. The cortex contains the pigment and determines hair's strength and elasticity.
12. The cuticle is the outermost layer, consisting of overlapping scales that protect the hair shaft.
13. Hair can stretch up to 30% of its original length when wet.
14. Human hair can be used to create wigs, hair extensions, and even art.
15. Hair has been used in forensic science to identify individuals through DNA analysis.
16. The average lifespan of a hair strand is 2 to 7 years.
17. Hair color can change naturally over time due to aging.
18. Hair loss can be caused by various factors, including genetics, hormones, and medical conditions.
19. The study of hair and its disorders is called trichology.
20. Hair on different parts of the body has varying growth rates and textures.
21. Hair on the head grows faster than hair on the rest of the body.
22. A single strand of hair can support up to 100 grams of weight.
23. Hair contains information about an individual's drug use history, as certain substances can be detected in hair follicles.
24. The world's longest recorded hair was over 18 feet (5.6 meters) long.
25. Hair can serve as a sensory organ, detecting movement and changes in the environment.
26. Some animals, like porcupines and hedgehogs, have modified hair called quills for defense.
27. Hair can trap air, providing insulation and helping to regulate body temperature.
28. In ancient Egypt, wigs and hairpieces were commonly worn as a status symbol.
29. Hair care products include shampoos, conditioners, hair sprays, and serums.
30. Split ends occur when the protective cuticle layer of hair is damaged.

31. Baldness, or alopecia, can be caused by genetics (male pattern baldness) or other factors.
32. The hormone dihydrotestosterone (DHT) is often linked to male pattern baldness.
33. Hair can be used for environmental purposes to monitor exposure to pollutants and toxins.
34. Some hair myths include that cutting your hair makes it grow faster (it doesn't) and that gray hair is caused by stress (it's primarily genetic).
35. The texture and appearance of hair can change due to factors like humidity and temperature.
36. Hair can be straightened or curled using various heat styling tools.
37. Braiding, weaving, and twisting are popular hair styling techniques in many cultures.
38. The pH of hair is typically around 4.5 to 5.5, making it slightly acidic.
39. Hair can become damaged from excessive heat styling, chemical treatments, and exposure to UV rays.
40. Hair loss can be temporary, as seen in conditions like telogen effluvium, which is often triggered by stress or illness.
41. Hair transplants involve moving hair follicles from one part of the body to another to treat baldness.
42. The smell of burning hair is distinctive and unpleasant due to the sulfur-containing compounds in keratin.
43. Hair follicles can become inflamed, leading to conditions like folliculitis.
44. Hair loss can also result from nutritional deficiencies, such as iron or biotin deficiency.
45. Hair is one of the fastest-growing tissues in the human body.
46. Hair color trends and preferences vary across cultures and time periods.
47. Hairs on the eyebrows and eyelashes have a shorter growth cycle compared to scalp hair.

48. The hair industry is a multibillion-dollar global market, encompassing products and services. Hair plays a significant role in self-expression and can be a source of personal identity and cultural significance.

49. In hair Transplant, hairs are extracted from occipital (Back of the head) because this area is resistant to DHT Hormone.

www.ingramcontent.com/pod-product-compliance
Lightning Source LLC
Chambersburg PA
CBHW041648150726
48005CB00015BB/2525